DR. BARBARA 3-DAY JUICE DETOX

Step by step guide to natural body cleansing and rejuvenate using nutritious and healthy recipes and smoothies for optimal health and vitality

Carlos Luz

Table of Contents

COPYRIGHT © 2023

All rights reserved. No part of this publication may be reproduced, distributed, or transmitted in any form or by any means, including photocopying, recording, or other electronic or mechanical methods, without the prior written permission of the publisher, except in the case of brief quotations embodied in critical reviews and certain other noncommercial uses permitted by copyright law.

CHAPTER ONE

Introduction to Dr. Barbara's Detox Method: Understanding the Benefits of Herbal Juicing for Cleansing

Juicing has gained significant popularity in recent years as a method for detoxification and cleansing. Among the myriad of juicing programs available, Dr. Barbara's Detox Method stands out for its emphasis on herbal ingredients and their purported health benefits. This comprehensive detox approach combines the power of various herbs and fruits to cleanse the body, boost energy levels, and promote overall well-being. In this detailed exploration, we will delve into the fundamentals of Dr. Barbara's Detox Method, uncovering its underlying principles, the benefits of herbal juicing for cleansing, and how it can contribute to a healthier lifestyle.

Understanding Detoxification:

Detoxification, often referred to as detox, is the process of eliminating toxins and harmful substances from the body. Our bodies naturally perform detoxification through organs like the liver, kidneys, and skin. However, due to factors such as poor dietary choices, environmental pollutants, and stress, our natural detoxification systems can become overwhelmed. This overload of toxins may lead to various health issues, including fatigue, digestive problems, and weakened immune function.

Dr. Barbara's Detox Method aims to support the body's natural detox processes by providing it with essential nutrients and antioxidants found in herbal juices. By consuming these nutrient-dense juices, individuals can help facilitate the removal of toxins from their bodies, promoting better health and vitality.

The Role of Herbal Juicing:

Herbal juicing involves extracting the juices from various herbs, vegetables, and fruits to create potent elixirs packed with vitamins, minerals, and phytonutrients. Unlike commercially processed juices, which often contain added sugars and preservatives, herbal juices are fresh, raw, and full of bioactive compounds that support health.

Dr. Barbara's Detox Method emphasizes the inclusion of specific herbs known for their detoxifying properties. These herbs may include dandelion root, cilantro, ginger, turmeric, and parsley, among others. Each herb offers unique benefits for cleansing and rejuvenating the body. For example, dandelion root is believed to support liver function, while cilantro may help remove heavy metals from the body. By combining these herbs in carefully crafted juice recipes, Dr. Barbara's Detox Method provides a comprehensive approach to detoxification.

Benefits of Herbal Juicing for Cleansing:

1. **Supports Liver Health:** The liver plays a crucial role in detoxification, filtering toxins from the bloodstream and breaking them down for elimination. Herbal juices rich in compounds like antioxidants and flavonoids can support liver function, enhancing its ability to detoxify the body.

2. **Promotes Digestive Health:** Many herbs used in Dr. Barbara's Detox Method possess digestive properties that can help alleviate bloating, gas, and constipation. Ingredients like ginger and mint may soothe the digestive tract, while fiber-rich fruits and vegetables support regular bowel movements.

3. **Boosts Energy Levels:** Detoxification can lead to increased energy levels as the body eliminates toxins that may contribute to fatigue and sluggishness. Herbal juices provide a concentrated source of nutrients that nourish the body at a cellular level, promoting vitality and well-being.

4. **Enhances Immune Function:** A healthy immune system is essential for defending the body against infections and illnesses. Herbal juices are rich in vitamins, minerals, and antioxidants that support immune function, helping to keep the body strong and resilient.

5. **Promotes Weight Loss:** Detoxification can aid in weight loss by removing excess waste and toxins from the body. Herbal

juices, particularly those with low sugar content and high fiber content, can support weight management goals by promoting satiety and reducing cravings for unhealthy foods.

How to Incorporate Dr. Barbara's Detox Method into Your Routine:

Incorporating Dr. Barbara's Detox Method into your routine is relatively straightforward, but it requires commitment and dedication. Here are some steps to get started:

1. **Consultation:** Before beginning any detox program, it's essential to consult with a healthcare professional, especially if you have any underlying health conditions or concerns. They can provide guidance tailored to your individual needs and ensure that detoxification is safe and appropriate for you.

2. **Preparation:** Prepare your body for detox by gradually reducing your intake of processed foods, caffeine, alcohol, and refined sugars. Focus on consuming whole, nutrient-dense foods to support your body's natural detoxification processes.

3. **Juice Recipes:** Experiment with different juice recipes provided by Dr. Barbara's Detox Method or create your own combinations using fresh herbs, vegetables, and fruits. Aim

for a variety of colors and flavors to ensure you're getting a wide range of nutrients.

4. **Hydration:** Stay hydrated throughout the detox process by drinking plenty of water in addition to herbal juices. Hydration is essential for flushing out toxins and supporting overall health.

5. **Mindful Eating:** Practice mindful eating during and after the detox program, paying attention to hunger cues and choosing nourishing foods that support your health goals. Focus on whole foods, such as fruits, vegetables, lean proteins, and healthy fats, to maintain the benefits of detoxification.

Conclusion:

Dr. Barbara's Detox Method offers a holistic approach to detoxification, harnessing the power of herbal juicing to cleanse the body, boost energy levels, and promote overall well-being. By understanding the benefits of herbal juicing for cleansing and incorporating this method into your routine, you can support your body's natural detoxification processes and embark on a path to better health. Remember to consult with a healthcare professional before beginning any detox program and listen to your body's signals throughout the process. With dedication and commitment, you can experience the transformative effects of

Dr. Barbara's Detox Method and enjoy renewed vitality and vitality.

CHAPTER TWO

The Importance of Detoxification: Exploring How Toxins Impact Health and Well-being

Detoxification is a crucial process that the body undergoes to eliminate harmful substances and toxins. In today's world, where we are exposed to an array of pollutants, chemicals, and stressors, the importance of effective detoxification cannot be overstated. This comprehensive exploration will delve into the significance of detoxification, elucidating how toxins impact health and well-being on multiple levels.

Understanding Toxins:

Toxins are substances that have the potential to cause harm to the body. They can be classified into two main categories: exogenous toxins, which originate from external sources such as pollutants, pesticides, and chemicals in food and water, and endogenous toxins, which are produced internally as byproducts of metabolic processes.

Exogenous toxins are ubiquitous in the environment, found in air pollution, contaminated water, processed foods, household cleaners, personal care products, and more. Endogenous toxins, on the other hand, include metabolic waste products like free radicals, excess hormones, and byproducts of cellular metabolism.

Impact of Toxins on Health and Well-being:

The accumulation of toxins in the body can have profound effects on health and well-being, impacting various systems and organs:

1. **Liver:** The liver is the body's primary detoxification organ, responsible for filtering toxins from the bloodstream and converting them into water-soluble compounds for elimination. Prolonged exposure to toxins can overwhelm the liver's detoxification pathways, leading to impaired liver function and the accumulation of toxins in the body.

2. **Digestive System:** Toxins can disrupt the balance of beneficial bacteria in the gut microbiome, leading to digestive issues such as bloating, gas, constipation, and diarrhea. An unhealthy gut microbiome can also compromise immune function and nutrient absorption, further exacerbating health problems.

3. **Immune System:** The immune system plays a crucial role in defending the body against pathogens and foreign invaders. However, exposure to toxins can weaken the immune system's response, making the body more susceptible to infections, allergies, and autoimmune disorders.

4. **Endocrine System:** Toxins known as endocrine disruptors can interfere with the normal function of hormones in the body, leading to hormonal imbalances and reproductive issues. Endocrine disruptors are found in various everyday

products, including plastics, pesticides, and personal care products.

5. **Nervous System:** Toxins can cross the blood-brain barrier and affect the central nervous system, leading to neurological symptoms such as headaches, brain fog, memory loss, and mood disorders. Heavy metals like lead, mercury, and aluminum are particularly damaging to the nervous system.

6. **Skin:** The skin is another important organ of detoxification, eliminating toxins through sweat. However, exposure to environmental toxins and harsh chemicals in personal care products can disrupt the skin's natural detoxification processes, leading to skin issues like acne, eczema, and premature aging.

The Importance of Detoxification:

Given the pervasive presence of toxins in our environment and their detrimental effects on health, effective detoxification is essential for maintaining overall well-being. Here are some reasons why detoxification is important:

1. **Enhanced Energy and Vitality:** By eliminating toxins from the body, detoxification can improve energy levels and promote vitality. Many people report feeling more energized and rejuvenated after completing a detox program.

2. **Supports Weight Management:** Toxins stored in fat cells can interfere with metabolism and contribute to weight gain. Detoxification can help release stored toxins and promote weight loss by optimizing metabolic function.

3. **Promotes Clearer Skin:** By removing toxins from the body, detoxification can improve skin health and promote a clearer complexion. Many individuals experience reduced acne, inflammation, and other skin issues after detoxifying.

4. **Boosts Immune Function:** A healthy immune system is essential for fighting off infections and illnesses. Detoxification supports immune function by reducing the burden of toxins on the body and promoting optimal immune response.

5. **Supports Longevity:** Chronic exposure to toxins is associated with an increased risk of chronic diseases such as cancer, cardiovascular disease, and neurodegenerative disorders. By reducing toxin exposure and supporting detoxification, individuals can promote longevity and reduce their risk of disease.

Methods of Detoxification:

There are various methods of detoxification, ranging from dietary changes and lifestyle modifications to specific detox programs and therapies. Some common methods include:

1. **Healthy Diet:** Eating a diet rich in whole, nutrient-dense foods can support detoxification by providing essential nutrients and antioxidants that support liver function and cellular health. Focus on organic fruits and vegetables, lean proteins, healthy fats, and plenty of water.

2. **Hydration:** Drinking an adequate amount of water is essential for flushing toxins from the body and supporting overall detoxification. Aim to drink at least eight glasses of water per day, and consider incorporating herbal teas and detoxifying drinks like lemon water and green tea.

3. **Herbal Supplements:** Certain herbs and botanicals have detoxifying properties that can support liver function, promote digestion, and enhance detoxification pathways. Milk thistle, dandelion root, turmeric, and cilantro are examples of herbs commonly used for detoxification.

4. **Sauna Therapy:** Sweating is another effective way to eliminate toxins from the body. Sauna therapy involves sitting in a sauna or steam room to induce sweating and promote detoxification through the skin.

5. **Colon Cleansing:** Colon cleansing therapies such as colon hydrotherapy or enemas can help remove impacted waste and toxins from the colon, promoting better digestive health and detoxification.

Conclusion:

In conclusion, detoxification is a critical process that plays a vital role in maintaining health and well-being in the face of environmental toxins and pollutants. By understanding the impact of toxins on the body and adopting effective detoxification strategies, individuals can support their body's natural detoxification processes and promote optimal health. Whether through dietary changes, lifestyle modifications, or specific detox programs, prioritizing detoxification can lead to increased energy, clearer skin, enhanced immune function, and a reduced risk of chronic disease.

CHAPTER THREE

Dr. Barbara's Philosophy on Herbal Juicing: Harnessing the Healing Power of Fresh, Nutrient-Dense Juices

Dr. Barbara's philosophy on herbal juicing revolves around the belief that fresh, nutrient-dense juices derived from herbs, vegetables, and fruits can serve as potent tools for healing and rejuvenation. With a focus on holistic health and natural remedies, Dr. Barbara emphasizes the importance of nourishing the body with essential nutrients while supporting its innate detoxification processes. In this comprehensive exploration, we will delve into the core principles of Dr. Barbara's philosophy on herbal juicing, examining how it harnesses the healing power of fresh juices to promote vitality and well-being.

Holistic Health Approach:

At the heart of Dr. Barbara's philosophy is a holistic approach to health, which recognizes the interconnectedness of the mind, body, and spirit. Rather than treating symptoms in isolation, holistic health focuses on addressing the root causes of imbalance and promoting overall wellness. Herbal juicing aligns perfectly with this approach by providing the body with a wide array of nutrients and bioactive compounds that support its natural healing mechanisms.

Dr. Barbara advocates for a whole-food, plant-based diet rich in fruits, vegetables, herbs, and spices, which are abundant sources of vitamins, minerals, antioxidants, and phytonutrients. By consuming fresh juices made from these nutrient-dense ingredients, individuals can nourish their bodies at a cellular level and support optimal health from the inside out.

The Healing Power of Fresh Juices:

Fresh juices are potent elixirs of health, packed with concentrated nutrients that are easily absorbed by the body. Unlike processed juices found in supermarkets, which are often laden with added sugars, preservatives, and artificial flavors, fresh juices contain only the pure essence of their ingredients, making them a powerhouse of nutrition.

Dr. Barbara believes that herbal juicing offers a convenient and effective way to flood the body with essential vitamins, minerals, and antioxidants, promoting detoxification, rejuvenation, and vitality. By harnessing the healing power of fresh juices, individuals can support their immune system, improve digestion, boost energy levels, and enhance overall well-being.

Supporting Detoxification:

Detoxification is a fundamental aspect of Dr. Barbara's philosophy on herbal juicing. The body's natural detoxification pathways, primarily facilitated by the liver, kidneys, and lymphatic system, can become overwhelmed by the constant exposure to environmental toxins, processed foods, and stress. Herbal juices provide a gentle yet effective means of supporting these detoxification processes, helping to eliminate accumulated toxins and restore balance to the body.

Many of the herbs and ingredients used in Dr. Barbara's juice recipes are specifically chosen for their detoxifying properties. For example, dandelion root is known for its ability to support liver function and aid in the elimination of toxins, while cilantro may help remove heavy metals from the body. By incorporating these detoxifying herbs into fresh juices, individuals can enhance their body's ability to cleanse and purify itself naturally.

Promoting Vitality and Well-being:

Ultimately, Dr. Barbara's philosophy on herbal juicing is rooted in the belief that optimal health is not merely the absence of disease but a state of vibrant vitality and well-being. By nourishing the body with fresh, nutrient-dense juices, individuals can support their body's natural healing processes, boost their immune system, increase energy levels, and experience greater vitality in all aspects of life.

In addition to physical health benefits, herbal juicing can also have profound effects on mental and emotional well-being. The abundance of vitamins, minerals, and antioxidants found in fresh juices can help reduce inflammation, support brain health, and improve mood, cognition, and overall mental clarity.

Conclusion:

Dr. Barbara's philosophy on herbal juicing embodies a holistic approach to health and wellness, emphasizing the healing power of fresh, nutrient-dense juices derived from herbs, vegetables, and fruits. By harnessing the natural goodness of these ingredients, individuals can support their body's detoxification processes, promote vitality and well-being, and experience a profound transformation in their health and quality of life. Whether as a daily wellness practice or a targeted detoxification program, herbal juicing offers a simple yet powerful way to nourish the body, mind, and spirit, paving the way for optimal health and vitality.

CHAPTER FOUR

Preparing for the Detox: Guidelines for Pre-Cleanse Preparation and Setting Intentions

Embarking on a detox journey requires thoughtful preparation and a clear intention to support the body's natural cleansing processes effectively. Preparing for the detox involves more than just adjusting your diet; it's about setting the stage for a transformative experience that nourishes not only your body but also your mind and spirit. In this comprehensive guide, we'll explore the essential guidelines for pre-cleanse preparation and setting intentions to maximize the benefits of your detox journey.

Understanding the Purpose of Pre-Cleanse Preparation:

Pre-cleanse preparation is a vital step in the detoxification process as it helps prime the body for the upcoming cleanse, reduces potential detox symptoms, and enhances the effectiveness of the detox protocol. The primary goals of pre-cleanse preparation include:

1. **Reducing Toxin Exposure:** Minimizing exposure to toxins from dietary and environmental sources helps lighten the detoxification burden on the body, allowing it to focus on eliminating stored toxins more efficiently.

2. **Supporting Detox Organs:** Preparing the liver, kidneys, and other detox organs through dietary and lifestyle adjustments helps optimize their function, ensuring a smoother detoxification process.

3. **Balancing Nutrient Intake:** Ensuring adequate intake of essential nutrients and hydration supports cellular function and helps prevent nutrient deficiencies during the cleanse.

Guidelines for Pre-Cleanse Preparation:

1. **Gradual Transition:** Begin transitioning to a cleaner diet at least one to two weeks before starting the detox. Gradually reduce or eliminate processed foods, refined sugars, caffeine, alcohol, and animal products while increasing your intake of fresh fruits, vegetables, whole grains, and plant-based proteins.

2. **Hydration:** Drink plenty of water throughout the day to stay hydrated and support the body's detoxification processes. Aim for at least eight glasses of water daily, and consider incorporating herbal teas and fresh juices for additional hydration.

3. **Reduce Toxin Exposure:** Minimize exposure to environmental toxins by choosing organic produce whenever possible, using natural and non-toxic household cleaners, and avoiding synthetic fragrances and personal care products containing harmful chemicals.

4. **Support Detox Organs:** Incorporate foods and supplements that support liver health, such as dandelion root, milk thistle, turmeric, and cruciferous vegetables like broccoli and kale. Include plenty of fiber-rich foods to support digestive health and regular elimination.

5. **Practice Mindful Eating:** Pay attention to your eating habits and cultivate mindful eating practices. Chew your food thoroughly, eat slowly, and savor each bite to enhance digestion and nutrient absorption.

6. **Reduce Stress:** Engage in stress-reducing activities such as yoga, meditation, deep breathing exercises, or spending time in nature to promote relaxation and support overall well-being.

Setting Intentions for the Detox:

Setting intentions is a powerful way to align your mind, body, and spirit with your detox goals and create a positive mindset for the journey ahead. Here are some tips for setting intentions for your detox:

1. **Clarify Your Intentions:** Take some time to reflect on why you're embarking on this detox journey. What are your goals? What do you hope to achieve? Clarifying your intentions will help guide your actions and keep you focused throughout the process.

2. **Visualize Success:** Visualize yourself completing the detox with ease and grace, feeling energized, rejuvenated, and empowered. Imagine the positive changes you'll experience in your health, energy levels, and overall well-being.

3. **Practice Gratitude:** Cultivate an attitude of gratitude for the opportunity to nourish and cleanse your body. Express gratitude for the abundance of fresh, wholesome foods available to support your health and vitality.

4. **Stay Present:** Stay present and mindful throughout the detox journey, focusing on each moment as it unfolds. Be open to the experiences, sensations, and insights that arise along the way, embracing them with curiosity and acceptance.

5. **Embrace Self-Compassion:** Be gentle and compassionate with yourself during the detox process. Honor your body's needs and listen to its cues without judgment or criticism. Celebrate your progress and acknowledge your efforts along the way.

Conclusion:

Preparing for a detox involves more than just changing your diet; it requires a holistic approach that addresses the needs of your body, mind, and spirit. By following the guidelines for pre-cleanse preparation and setting intentions for the detox journey, you can create a supportive environment that maximizes the benefits of the cleanse and fosters a deeper sense of well-being. Remember to approach the detox with an open mind and heart, embracing the opportunity for growth, healing, and transformation. With dedication, mindfulness, and self-care, you can embark on your detox journey with confidence and clarity, knowing that you're taking proactive steps towards optimal health and vitality.

CHAPTER FIVE

The 3-Day Herbal Juice Detox Protocol: Step-by-Step Instructions for Daily Juicing and Hydration

Embarking on a 3-day herbal juice detox offers a rejuvenating opportunity to cleanse your body, boost energy levels, and promote overall well-being. This comprehensive guide provides step-by-step instructions for daily juicing and hydration during the detox period, ensuring a smooth and effective cleansing experience.

Day 1: Preparation and Setting Intentions

1. **Morning Ritual:** Start your day with a glass of warm lemon water to hydrate the body and support digestion. Take a few moments for quiet reflection or meditation to set positive intentions for the detox journey ahead.

2. **Preparation:** Review the juice recipes and ingredients for the day. Ensure you have all the necessary herbs, vegetables, and fruits on hand. Wash and prepare the produce as needed.

3. **Hydration:** Throughout the day, drink plenty of water between juices to stay hydrated and support the body's detoxification processes. Aim for at least 8-10 glasses of

water, herbal teas, or infused water with lemon and cucumber.

4. **Juice Recipes:** Follow the provided juice recipes for each meal and snack time. Incorporate a variety of herbs, vegetables, and fruits known for their detoxifying properties, such as dandelion greens, parsley, ginger, turmeric, kale, celery, cucumber, lemon, and apple.

5. **Meal Schedule:** Plan your meals and snacks according to the recommended schedule, spacing them out evenly throughout the day to maintain stable blood sugar levels and energy levels.

6. **Mindful Eating:** Practice mindful eating by savoring each sip of juice and paying attention to how it nourishes your body. Take breaks between meals to rest, relax, and recharge.

7. **Evening Reflection:** At the end of the day, take a moment to reflect on your experiences during the detox. Notice any physical, emotional, or mental changes and express gratitude for the opportunity to nourish and cleanse your body.

Day 2: Deepening the Cleanse

1. **Morning Routine:** Begin your day with a gentle stretching or yoga session to awaken the body and promote circulation.

Follow with a refreshing glass of cucumber or celery juice to hydrate and alkalize the body.

2. **Hydration:** Continue to prioritize hydration throughout the day, alternating between herbal teas, water, and fresh juices. Experiment with different herbal infusions, such as mint, chamomile, or nettle, to support detoxification and relaxation.

3. **Juice Recipes:** Explore new juice combinations and flavors to keep your taste buds engaged and satisfied. Consider incorporating detoxifying herbs like cilantro, mint, and basil into your juices for added flavor and benefits.

4. **Physical Activity:** Engage in light physical activity or movement throughout the day, such as walking, yoga, or stretching, to support lymphatic drainage and circulation. Listen to your body and avoid strenuous exercise during the detox period.

5. **Rest and Relaxation:** Take breaks as needed to rest, relax, and rejuvenate your body and mind. Consider incorporating stress-reducing activities like meditation, deep breathing exercises, or gentle massage to promote relaxation and well-being.

6. **Evening Ritual:** Wind down in the evening with a calming herbal tea or warm almond milk infused with cinnamon and

nutmeg. Reflect on the day's experiences and express gratitude for the nourishment and healing provided by the detox protocol.

Day 3: Integration and Transition

1. **Morning Ritual:** Start your day with a sense of gratitude and appreciation for the journey you've embarked on. Take a moment to visualize yourself completing the detox with ease and grace, feeling renewed and revitalized.

2. **Hydration:** Continue to prioritize hydration on the final day of the detox, focusing on replenishing electrolytes and supporting optimal hydration levels. Consider adding a pinch of Himalayan salt to your water or juices to support electrolyte balance.

3. **Reflection and Integration:** Reflect on the insights and experiences gained during the detox journey. Notice any changes in your energy levels, digestion, mood, and overall well-being. Take note of any habits or patterns you'd like to carry forward beyond the cleanse.

4. **Transitioning Out:** As you transition out of the detox, gradually reintroduce solid foods into your diet, starting with light, easy-to-digest meals such as steamed vegetables, soups, and salads. Chew your food thoroughly and pay attention to how your body responds to different foods.

5. **Celebration:** Celebrate the completion of your 3-day herbal juice detox with a sense of accomplishment and pride. Acknowledge the dedication and commitment you've shown to your health and well-being, and carry forward the lessons learned into your daily life.

6. **Continued Wellness:** Incorporate the principles of mindful eating, hydration, and self-care into your daily routine to support ongoing health and vitality. Consider incorporating regular juice days or mini-detoxes into your routine as a way to reset and rejuvenate periodically.

Embarking on a 3-day herbal juice detox can be a transformative experience that revitalizes your body, mind, and spirit. By following the step-by-step instructions provided in this guide, you can navigate the detox process with ease and confidence, maximizing the benefits of the cleanse and promoting overall well-being. Remember to approach the detox with an open mind and heart, embracing the opportunity for growth, healing, and renewal. With dedication, mindfulness, and self-care, you can emerge from the detox feeling refreshed, rejuvenated, and ready to embrace a healthier, more vibrant life.

DR. BARBARA 3-DAY JUICE DETOX PLAN FOR FULL-BODY DETOX

Day 1

Morning

Green Detox Juice

- 2 cups spinach
- 1 cucumber
- 2 celery stalks
- 1 green apple
- 1 lemon (peeled)
- 1-inch ginger root

Blend or juice all ingredients together. Drink immediately.

Mid-Morning

Citrus Cleanser

- 2 oranges
- 1 grapefruit
- 1 lemon
- 1 lime

Juice all ingredients together. Drink immediately.

Lunch

Carrot-Apple-Ginger Juice

- 4 carrots

- 2 apples

- 1-inch ginger root

Juice all ingredients together. Drink immediately.

Afternoon

Beet Detox Juice

- 2 beets

- 2 carrots

- 1 apple

- 1 lemon (peeled)

Juice all ingredients together. Drink immediately.

Dinner

Pineapple Mint Juice

- 1/2 pineapple

- 1 cucumber

- 1/2 lemon (peeled)

- Handful of mint leaves

Juice all ingredients together. Drink immediately.

Day 2

Morning

Green Apple Lemonade

- 2 green apples
- 1 lemon (peeled)
- 1 cucumber
- Handful of kale

Juice all ingredients together. Drink immediately.

Mid-Morning

Ginger Citrus Juice

- 3 oranges
- 1-inch ginger root
- 1 lemon

Juice all ingredients together. Drink immediately.

Lunch

Tomato-Veggie Juice

- 3 tomatoes

- 1 cucumber

- 1 celery stalk

- Handful of parsley

- 1 lemon (peeled)

Juice all ingredients together. Drink immediately.

Afternoon

Watermelon Mint Juice

- 2 cups watermelon

- 1/2 lime

- Handful of mint leaves

Juice all ingredients together. Drink immediately.

Dinner

Sweet Potato Juice

- 1 sweet potato

- 2 carrots

- 1 apple

Juice all ingredients together. Drink immediately.

Day 3

Morning

Tropical Green Juice

- 2 cups spinach
- 1/2 pineapple
- 1/2 cucumber
- 1 lime

Juice all ingredients together. Drink immediately.

Mid-Morning

Blueberry Detox Juice

- 1 cup blueberries
- 1 apple
- 1/2 lemon (peeled)
- 1 cucumber

Juice all ingredients together. Drink immediately.

Lunch

Celery Cleanser Juice

- 4 celery stalks

- 2 green apples

- 1 cucumber

- 1 lemon

Juice all ingredients together. Drink immediately.

Afternoon

Berry Beet Juice

- 2 beets

- 1 cup strawberries

- 1 apple

- 1/2 lemon (peeled)

Juice all ingredients together. Drink immediately.

Dinner

Mango Carrot Juice

- 2 carrots

- 1 mango

- 1 orange

Juice all ingredients together. Drink immediately.

Additional Tips:

- **Stay Hydrated**: Drink plenty of water throughout the day.

- **Listen to Your Body**: If you feel hungry, add more juices or incorporate a small, healthy snack like a handful of nuts or a piece of fruit.

- **Rest**: Ensure you get enough sleep each night to support the detox process.

This 3-day detox plan focuses on providing your body with essential vitamins, minerals, and antioxidants while giving your digestive system a break. Enjoy the refreshing flavors and the benefits of a rejuvenated body!

CHAPTER SIX

Selecting the Right Herbs: Identifying Key Ingredients for Detoxifying Herbal Juices

Choosing the appropriate herbs is essential for creating effective detoxifying herbal juices. Each herb possesses unique properties that support the body's natural detoxification processes, making them valuable additions to your juice recipes. In this guide, we'll explore key ingredients for detoxifying herbal juices and provide insights into their benefits and uses.

Dandelion Root:

Dandelion root is renowned for its liver-cleansing properties, making it a staple ingredient in detoxifying herbal juices. Rich in antioxidants and phytonutrients, dandelion root supports liver function by promoting bile production and enhancing detoxification pathways. Additionally, dandelion root has diuretic properties that aid in the elimination of toxins through the urinary system.

Milk Thistle:

Milk thistle is another potent herb that supports liver health and detoxification. The active compound in milk thistle, silymarin, has been shown to protect liver cells from damage and promote regeneration. Incorporating milk thistle into your herbal juices can help support liver function and protect against the harmful effects of toxins and free radicals.

Turmeric:

Turmeric is well-known for its anti-inflammatory and antioxidant properties, making it a valuable addition to detoxifying herbal juices. Curcumin, the active compound in turmeric, has been shown to support liver function, enhance detoxification, and reduce inflammation throughout the body. Adding turmeric to your juices can help promote overall health and well-being.

Ginger:

Ginger is a versatile herb with powerful detoxifying properties. It aids digestion, promotes circulation, and supports detoxification pathways in the body. Ginger also has anti-inflammatory and antioxidant effects, making it beneficial for overall health and well-being. Incorporating fresh ginger into your herbal juices can help enhance their detoxifying effects and promote digestive health.

Cilantro:

Cilantro is known for its ability to help remove heavy metals and other toxins from the body. It contains compounds that bind to heavy metals and facilitate their elimination through urine and feces. Including cilantro in your herbal juices can support detoxification and promote overall health and vitality.

Parsley:

Parsley is rich in chlorophyll, vitamins, minerals, and antioxidants that support detoxification and promote overall health. It has diuretic properties that help flush out toxins from the body and support kidney function. Adding parsley to your herbal juices can help cleanse the body and support optimal health and well-being.

Nettle Leaf:

Nettle leaf is a nutrient-dense herb that supports detoxification and promotes overall health and vitality. It is rich in vitamins, minerals, and antioxidants that support liver function and enhance detoxification pathways. Nettle leaf also has diuretic properties that aid in the elimination of toxins from the body.

Burdock Root:

Burdock root is a traditional herb used for its detoxifying properties. It supports liver function, promotes digestion, and enhances the elimination of toxins from the body. Burdock root is also rich in antioxidants that help protect against oxidative stress and promote overall health and well-being.

Lemon:

Lemon is a cleansing and alkalizing fruit that adds a refreshing flavor to herbal juices. It is rich in vitamin C, antioxidants, and bioflavonoids that support liver function and promote detoxification. Lemon also stimulates digestion and helps balance pH levels in the body, making it an excellent addition to detoxifying herbal juices.

Conclusion:

Selecting the right herbs is crucial for creating effective detoxifying herbal juices. Each herb offers unique properties that support the body's natural detoxification processes and promote overall health and well-being. By incorporating a variety of detoxifying herbs into your juice recipes, you can create potent elixirs that cleanse, nourish, and rejuvenate your body from the inside out. Experiment with different combinations of herbs to find the flavors and benefits that resonate with you, and enjoy the transformative effects of detoxifying herbal juices on your health and vitality.

CHAPTER SEVEN

Supporting the Body's Elimination Pathways: Understanding How Juicing Enhances Detox Processes

Juicing plays a significant role in supporting the body's natural detoxification processes by providing essential nutrients, antioxidants, and hydration that facilitate the elimination of toxins. Understanding how juicing enhances detox processes involves recognizing the various ways in which fresh juices support the body's elimination pathways, including the liver, kidneys, digestive system, skin, and lymphatic system.

Liver Support:

The liver is the body's primary detoxification organ, responsible for filtering toxins from the bloodstream and converting them into less harmful substances for elimination. Juicing supports liver function by providing a concentrated source of nutrients and antioxidants that support detoxification pathways. Ingredients like dandelion root, milk thistle, turmeric, and ginger are particularly beneficial for liver health and can help enhance the liver's ability to neutralize toxins and remove them from the body.

Kidney Support:

The kidneys play a crucial role in filtering waste products and toxins from the blood and excreting them through urine. Juicing supports kidney function by providing hydration and essential nutrients that support urinary health and promote the elimination of toxins. Ingredients like cucumber, celery, parsley, and lemon are diuretic and help flush toxins from the body by increasing urine production and supporting kidney function.

Digestive Support:

The digestive system plays a vital role in detoxification by breaking down food, absorbing nutrients, and eliminating waste products. Juicing supports digestive health by providing easily digestible nutrients and fiber that promote regular bowel movements and support the elimination of toxins through the stool. Ingredients like leafy greens, apples, ginger, and lemon help promote digestion, alleviate bloating and gas, and support a healthy gut microbiome.

Skin Support:

The skin is the body's largest organ of elimination, responsible for excreting toxins through sweat. Juicing supports skin health by providing hydration and antioxidants that promote detoxification and reduce inflammation. Ingredients like cucumber, celery, lemon, and leafy greens help hydrate the skin, support lymphatic drainage, and promote a clear complexion.

Lymphatic Support:

The lymphatic system plays a crucial role in detoxification by transporting toxins and waste products away from tissues and organs and excreting them through lymphatic vessels. Juicing supports lymphatic drainage by providing hydration and nutrients that support lymphatic circulation and promote the elimination of toxins. Ingredients like leafy greens, parsley, cilantro, and lemon help support lymphatic function and promote detoxification.

Antioxidant Support:

Antioxidants are compounds that neutralize free radicals and protect cells from oxidative damage caused by toxins and environmental stressors. Juicing is rich in antioxidants from fruits, vegetables, and herbs, which help support cellular health and enhance detoxification processes. Ingredients like berries, leafy greens, turmeric, and ginger are particularly rich in antioxidants and help protect against oxidative stress and inflammation.

Conclusion:

Juicing enhances the body's natural detoxification processes by supporting the liver, kidneys, digestive system, skin, and lymphatic system. By providing hydration, essential nutrients, antioxidants, and fiber, fresh juices help facilitate the elimination of toxins and promote overall health and well-being. Incorporating a variety of detoxifying ingredients into your juice recipes can help optimize detox processes and support your body's ability to cleanse and rejuvenate from the inside out.

CHAPTER EIGHT

Detoxification Symptoms and Side Effects: Managing Potential Reactions During the Cleanse

Embarking on a detoxification cleanse can trigger a range of symptoms and side effects as the body releases stored toxins and adjusts to dietary and lifestyle changes. Understanding and effectively managing these potential reactions are essential for a safe and successful cleanse experience. In this guide, we'll explore common detoxification symptoms and side effects and provide strategies for managing them to ensure a smooth and comfortable cleanse journey.

Common Detoxification Symptoms:

1. **Fatigue:** Fatigue is a common symptom during detoxification as the body redirects energy towards cleansing and healing processes. You may experience feelings of tiredness, lethargy, or low energy levels, especially in the initial days of the cleanse.

2. **Headaches:** Headaches can occur as the body eliminates toxins, particularly if you're reducing caffeine intake or experiencing caffeine withdrawal. Dehydration and changes in blood sugar levels can also contribute to headaches during the cleanse.

3. **Digestive Issues:** Digestive issues such as bloating, gas, constipation, or diarrhea may arise as the body adjusts to dietary changes and eliminates toxins. Increased fiber intake from fruits, vegetables, and herbs in juices can stimulate bowel movements and promote detoxification.

4. **Skin Breakouts:** Skin breakouts, acne flare-ups, or rashes may occur as the body eliminates toxins through the skin. This is a common detoxification response as the skin works to expel impurities and restore balance.

5. **Mood Changes:** Mood changes, irritability, or emotional fluctuations can occur as the body releases stored toxins and undergoes biochemical changes. Hormonal imbalances, stress, and changes in neurotransmitter levels may contribute to mood swings during the cleanse.

6. **Flu-like Symptoms:** Flu-like symptoms such as body aches, chills, and mild fever may occur as the body detoxifies and eliminates pathogens and toxins. These symptoms are usually transient and indicate that the body is actively cleansing.

Strategies for Managing Detoxification Symptoms:

1. **Stay Hydrated:** Drink plenty of water, herbal teas, and fresh juices throughout the cleanse to stay hydrated and support

detoxification processes. Hydration helps flush out toxins and alleviate symptoms like fatigue, headaches, and digestive issues.

2. **Gradual Transition:** Ease into the cleanse by gradually reducing caffeine, sugar, processed foods, and animal products in the days leading up to the cleanse. This can help minimize withdrawal symptoms and support a smoother transition.

3. **Rest and Relaxation:** Prioritize rest and relaxation during the cleanse to support the body's healing processes. Engage in gentle activities like yoga, meditation, deep breathing exercises, or gentle stretching to promote relaxation and stress relief.

4. **Support Detox Organs:** Incorporate foods and herbs that support liver and kidney health, such as dandelion root, milk thistle, turmeric, ginger, and parsley. These ingredients help enhance detoxification pathways and support the body's natural cleansing mechanisms.

5. **Manage Stress:** Practice stress management techniques such as mindfulness, meditation, journaling, or spending time in nature to reduce stress levels and promote emotional well-being during the cleanse. Stress reduction supports detoxification and overall health.

6. **Listen to Your Body:** Pay attention to your body's signals and adjust your cleanse accordingly. If you experience severe or prolonged symptoms, consider modifying your cleanse or seeking guidance from a healthcare professional.

7. **Post-cleanse Transition:** Gradually reintroduce solid foods into your diet after the cleanse, starting with light, easily digestible meals. Focus on whole, nutrient-dense foods like fruits, vegetables, whole grains, and lean proteins to support ongoing detoxification and maintain the benefits of the cleanse.

Conclusion:

Detoxification symptoms and side effects are common as the body undergoes cleansing and adjustment during a cleanse. By understanding these potential reactions and implementing strategies to manage them effectively, you can navigate the cleanse journey with greater ease and comfort. Remember to prioritize hydration, rest, nourishing foods, and stress management techniques to support your body's natural detoxification processes and promote overall health and well-being. If you have any concerns or experience severe symptoms during the cleanse, consult with a healthcare professional for personalized guidance and support.

CHAPTER NINE

Testimonials of Transformation: Inspiring Stories of Individuals Who Have Completed Dr. Barbara's 3-Day Herbal Juice Detox

Embarking on Dr. Barbara's 3-Day Herbal Juice Detox can be a transformative experience, leading to renewed vitality, improved well-being, and a deeper connection with one's body. Through the stories of individuals who have completed the detox, we gain insight into the profound impact it can have on physical health, mental clarity, and overall quality of life. Here are inspiring testimonials of transformation from individuals who have experienced the benefits of Dr. Barbara's herbal juice cleanse:

1. Sarah's Journey to Renewed Energy and Vitality:

"After years of feeling sluggish and lethargic, I decided to try Dr. Barbara's 3-Day Herbal Juice Detox. The results were nothing short of remarkable. By the end of the cleanse, I felt lighter, more energized, and clearer-headed than I had in years. My digestion improved, my skin cleared up, and I felt a renewed sense of vitality that I hadn't experienced in a long time. Dr. Barbara's detox was a game-changer for me, and I'm grateful for the opportunity to reclaim my health and well-being."

2. Mark's Experience of Mental Clarity and Focus:

"As someone who struggles with brain fog and lack of focus, I was intrigued by the potential cognitive benefits of Dr. Barbara's herbal juice cleanse. I decided to give it a try, and I was amazed by the results. By the second day of the cleanse, my mind felt clearer, sharper, and more focused than it had in years. I was able to concentrate better at work, and my productivity soared. The detox not only cleansed my body but also revitalized my mind, leaving me feeling more alert, present, and engaged in life."

3. Emily's Journey to Radiant Skin and Inner Glow:

"I've always struggled with acne-prone skin and tried countless skincare products with little success. Desperate for a solution, I decided to try Dr. Barbara's 3-Day Herbal Juice Detox as a natural approach to clear skin. To my delight, the results were astonishing. Within days of starting the cleanse, my skin began to clear up, and by the end of the detox, my complexion was radiant and glowing. Not only did the detox improve my skin, but it also gave me a newfound sense of confidence and self-esteem. Dr. Barbara's cleanse has truly transformed my skin and my life."

4. David's Journey to Weight Loss and Improved Digestion:

"After years of struggling with excess weight and digestive issues, I knew I needed to make a change. Dr. Barbara's 3-Day Herbal Juice Detox provided the reset my body desperately needed. Not only did I shed a few pounds during the cleanse, but I also experienced significant improvements in my digestion. Bloating, gas, and indigestion became a thing of the past, and I felt lighter and more comfortable in my body. The detox kick-started my journey to better health, and I'm grateful for the lasting impact it has had on my weight and digestion."

5. Rachel's Experience of Emotional Balance and Well-being:

"As someone who struggles with anxiety and stress, I was drawn to the emotional benefits of Dr. Barbara's herbal juice cleanse. The cleanse provided a much-needed opportunity for self-care and introspection, allowing me to slow down, reconnect with my body, and nourish myself from the inside out. By the end of the detox, I felt a profound sense of calm, balance, and inner peace that I hadn't experienced in years. Dr. Barbara's cleanse has helped me cultivate greater emotional resilience and well-being, and I'm grateful for the journey of self-discovery it has facilitated."

Conclusion:

These testimonials offer a glimpse into the transformative power of Dr. Barbara's 3-Day Herbal Juice Detox, showcasing the diverse benefits it can have on physical health, mental clarity, emotional well-being, and overall quality of life. From renewed energy and vitality to clearer skin and improved digestion, individuals who have completed the cleanse have experienced profound transformations that have positively impacted every aspect of their lives. Whether seeking to reclaim health, revitalize the mind, or cultivate inner peace, Dr. Barbara's herbal juice cleanse offers a path to holistic wellness and a renewed sense of vitality.

CHAPTER TEN

Post-Detox Maintenance: Strategies for Transitioning Back to Solid Foods and Sustaining Healthful Habits

Completing a detoxification cleanse marks an important milestone in your wellness journey, but it's equally essential to maintain the benefits and continue supporting your health after the cleanse. Transitioning back to solid foods and sustaining healthful habits are crucial aspects of post-detox maintenance. In this guide, we'll explore strategies for transitioning back to solid foods and implementing sustainable habits to support long-term health and well-being.

1. Gradual Reintroduction of Solid Foods:

After completing a detox cleanse, it's essential to reintroduce solid foods gradually to avoid overwhelming your digestive system. Start with light, easily digestible foods such as steamed vegetables, soups, salads, and whole grains. Incorporate whole, nutrient-dense foods gradually, paying attention to how your body responds to different foods.

2. Emphasize Whole, Plant-Based Foods:

Focus on incorporating a variety of whole, plant-based foods into your diet to support ongoing health and vitality. Load up on fruits, vegetables, legumes, whole grains, nuts, seeds, and healthy fats to provide your body with essential nutrients, fiber, and antioxidants. Aim to fill your plate with colorful, nutrient-rich foods to support overall health and well-being.

3. Mindful Eating Practices:

Practice mindful eating to cultivate a deeper connection with your body's hunger and fullness cues and enhance digestion. Eat slowly, chew your food thoroughly, and savor each bite to promote better digestion and nutrient absorption. Pay attention to how different foods make you feel and adjust your diet accordingly to support your body's needs.

4. Hydration and Fluid Intake:

Continue prioritizing hydration by drinking plenty of water, herbal teas, and fresh juices throughout the day. Staying hydrated supports detoxification, aids digestion, and promotes overall health and well-being. Aim to drink at least eight glasses of water daily and incorporate hydrating foods like fruits and vegetables into your diet.

5. Maintain a Balanced Diet:

Focus on maintaining a balanced diet that includes a variety of macronutrients, micronutrients, and phytonutrients to support optimal health. Include a mix of carbohydrates, proteins, and healthy fats in your meals, along with a diverse range of fruits, vegetables, and whole grains. Listen to your body's hunger and satiety signals and adjust your portion sizes accordingly.

6. Regular Physical Activity:

Stay active and incorporate regular physical activity into your daily routine to support overall health and well-being. Engage in activities you enjoy, such as walking, jogging, yoga, swimming, or strength training, to promote cardiovascular health, muscle strength, flexibility, and mental well-being. Aim for at least 30 minutes of moderate-intensity exercise most days of the week.

7. Prioritize Sleep and Stress Management:

Make sleep and stress management a priority to support optimal health and well-being. Aim for seven to nine hours of quality sleep each night to promote rest and recovery. Practice stress-reducing techniques such as meditation, deep breathing exercises, mindfulness, or spending time in nature to promote relaxation and resilience.

8. Cultivate Healthy Habits:

Focus on cultivating healthy habits that support your physical, mental, and emotional well-being. This may include meal planning, batch cooking, mindful eating, regular exercise, adequate sleep, stress management, and self-care practices. Consistency is key to sustaining healthful habits over the long term.

Conclusion:

Transitioning back to solid foods and sustaining healthful habits after completing a detox cleanse is essential for maintaining the benefits and supporting long-term health and well-being. By gradually reintroducing solid foods, emphasizing whole, plant-based foods, practicing mindful eating, staying hydrated, maintaining a balanced diet, engaging in regular physical activity, prioritizing sleep and stress management, and cultivating healthy habits, you can support your body's ongoing detoxification processes and promote optimal health and vitality for years to come. Remember to listen to your body, honor its needs, and make choices that support your overall well-being on your wellness journey.

Tila:

Definition: Tila, also known as linden flower or lime blossom, refers to the flowers of the Tilia genus, primarily Tilia europaea and Tilia cordata. These trees are native to Europe, but they are also cultivated in other regions for their fragrant and medicinal flowers.

Ingredients: Tila flowers contain various bioactive compounds, including flavonoids, phenolic acids, and volatile oils. These compounds are believed to contribute to the herb's medicinal properties, including its potential as a mild sedative, anxiolytic, and anti-inflammatory agent.

How to Prepare: Tila flowers are typically prepared and consumed as an herbal tea or infusion. To make tea, dried tila flowers are steeped in hot water for several minutes before being strained and consumed.

Dosage: The appropriate dosage of tila can vary depending on factors such as age, health status, and the specific preparation being used. It's important to follow the recommended dosage on the product label or consult with a qualified herbalist or healthcare professional for personalized guidance.

How to Use: Tila tea is typically taken orally. It's often consumed in the evening as a calming bedtime beverage or during times of stress or anxiety. It's important to use tila products as directed and to discontinue use if any adverse effects occur.

Side Effects: Tila is generally considered safe for most people when used in moderate amounts. However, some individuals may experience allergic reactions or digestive upset. It may also interact with certain medications or have adverse effects in individuals with certain health conditions. It's important to use tila under the guidance of a healthcare professional and to discontinue use if any adverse effects occur.

Valerian:

Definition: Valerian, scientifically known as Valeriana officinalis, is a perennial flowering plant native to Europe and Asia. It has been used for centuries in traditional medicine for its potential calming and sedative effects.

Ingredients: Valerian root contains several bioactive compounds, including valerenic acid, valepotriates, and volatile oils. These compounds are believed to contribute to the herb's medicinal properties, including its potential as a sedative, anxiolytic, and sleep aid.

How to Prepare: Valerian root is typically prepared and consumed as an herbal tea, tincture, or capsule. To make tea, dried valerian root is steeped in hot water for several minutes before being strained and consumed. Tinctures are prepared by steeping the root in alcohol or vinegar to extract its active compounds.

Dosage: The appropriate dosage of valerian can vary depending on factors such as age, health status, and the specific preparation being used. It's important to follow the recommended dosage on the product label or consult with a qualified herbalist or healthcare professional for personalized guidance.

How to Use: Valerian tea, tincture, or capsules are typically taken orally. It's often consumed in the evening as a sleep aid or during times of stress or anxiety. It's important to use valerian products as directed and to discontinue use if any adverse effects occur.

Side Effects: Valerian is generally considered safe for most people when used in moderate amounts. However, some individuals may experience mild side effects such as drowsiness, headache, or gastrointestinal upset. It may also interact with certain medications or have adverse effects in individuals with certain health conditions. It's important to use valerian under the guidance of a healthcare professional and to discontinue use if any adverse effects occur.

Wild Cherry Bark:

Definition: Wild cherry bark, scientifically known as Prunus serotina, is the bark obtained from the black cherry tree native to North America. It has been used traditionally in Native American and folk medicine for its potential health benefits, particularly for respiratory and digestive issues.

Ingredients: Wild cherry bark contains various bioactive compounds, including cyanogenic glycosides (such as prunasin and amygdalin), flavonoids, and phenolic acids. These compounds are believed to contribute to the herb's medicinal properties, including its potential as an expectorant, cough suppressant, and mild sedative.

How to Prepare: Wild cherry bark is typically prepared and consumed as an herbal tea, decoction, or syrup. To make tea, dried wild cherry bark is steeped in hot water for several minutes before being strained and consumed. Decoctions involve boiling the bark in water to extract its active compounds, while syrups are made by simmering the bark with sugar or honey to create a thick, sweet liquid.

Dosage: The appropriate dosage of wild cherry bark can vary depending on factors such as age, health status, and the specific preparation being used. It's important to follow the recommended dosage on the product label or consult with a qualified herbalist or healthcare professional for personalized guidance.

How to Use: Wild cherry bark tea, decoction, or syrup is typically taken orally. It's often consumed to soothe coughs, sore throats, and other respiratory symptoms. It's important to use wild cherry bark products as directed and to discontinue use if any adverse effects occur.

Side Effects: Wild cherry bark is generally considered safe for most people when used in moderate amounts. However, it contains cyanogenic glycosides, which can release cyanide in the body when metabolized. While the risk of cyanide poisoning from consuming wild cherry bark is low when used appropriately, excessive intake or prolonged use may lead to adverse effects. It's important to use wild cherry bark under the guidance of a healthcare professional and to discontinue use if any adverse effects occur.

Yellowdock:

Definition: Yellowdock, scientifically known as Rumex crispus, is a perennial flowering plant native to Europe and western Asia but is also found in North America. It has a long history of use in traditional medicine, particularly among Indigenous peoples, for its potential health benefits.

Ingredients: Yellowdock root contains various bioactive compounds, including anthraquinone glycosides (such as emodin and chrysophanol), tannins, and vitamins (including vitamin A and vitamin C). These compounds are believed to contribute to the herb's medicinal properties, including its potential as a laxative, blood cleanser, and liver tonic.

How to Prepare: Yellowdock root is typically prepared and consumed as an herbal tea, tincture, or capsule. To make tea, dried yellowdock root is steeped in hot water for several minutes before being strained and consumed. Tinctures are prepared by steeping the root in alcohol or vinegar to extract its active compounds.

Dosage: The appropriate dosage of yellowdock can vary depending on factors such as age, health status, and the specific preparation being used. It's important to follow the recommended dosage on the product label or consult with a qualified herbalist or healthcare professional for personalized guidance.

How to Use: Yellowdock tea, tincture, or capsules are typically taken orally. It's often consumed to support digestion, promote bowel regularity, and cleanse the blood. It's important to use yellowdock products as directed and to discontinue use if any adverse effects occur.

Side Effects: Yellowdock is generally considered safe for most people when used in moderate amounts. However, some individuals may experience mild side effects such as gastrointestinal upset or allergic reactions. It may also interact with certain medications or have adverse effects in individuals with certain health conditions. It's important to use yellowdock under the guidance of a healthcare professional and to discontinue use if any adverse effects occur.

Yellowdock Root:

Definition: Yellowdock root, scientifically known as Rumex crispus, is the root of a perennial flowering plant native to Europe and western Asia, also found in North America. It has a long history of use in traditional medicine, particularly among Indigenous peoples, for its potential health benefits.

Ingredients: Yellowdock root contains various bioactive compounds, including anthraquinone glycosides (such as emodin and chrysophanol), tannins, and vitamins (including vitamin A and vitamin C). These compounds are believed to contribute to the herb's medicinal properties, including its potential as a laxative, blood cleanser, and liver tonic.

How to Prepare: Yellowdock root is typically prepared and consumed as an herbal tea, tincture, or capsule. To make tea, dried yellowdock root is steeped in hot water for several minutes before being strained and consumed. Tinctures are prepared by steeping the root in alcohol or vinegar to extract its active compounds.

Dosage: The appropriate dosage of yellowdock root can vary depending on factors such as age, health status, and the specific preparation being used. It's important to follow the recommended dosage on the product label or consult with a qualified herbalist or healthcare professional for personalized guidance.

How to Use: Yellowdock root tea, tincture, or capsules are typically taken orally. It's often consumed to support digestion, promote bowel regularity, and cleanse the blood. It's important to use yellowdock root products as directed and to discontinue use if any adverse effects occur.

Side Effects: Yellowdock root is generally considered safe for most people when used in moderate amounts. However, some individuals may experience mild side effects such as gastrointestinal upset or allergic reactions. It may also interact with certain medications or have adverse effects in individuals with certain health conditions. It's important to use yellowdock root under the guidance of a healthcare professional and to discontinue use if any adverse effects occur.

Agrimony:

Definition: Agrimony, scientifically known as Agrimonia eupatoria, is a perennial herbaceous plant native to Europe, Asia, and North America. It has a long history of use in traditional medicine, particularly in European folk medicine, for its potential health benefits.

Ingredients: Agrimony contains various bioactive compounds, including tannins, flavonoids, phenolic acids, and volatile oils. These compounds are believed to contribute to the herb's medicinal properties, including its potential as an astringent, anti-inflammatory, and digestive aid.

How to Prepare: Agrimony is typically prepared and consumed as an herbal tea, tincture, or poultice. To make tea, dried agrimony leaves and flowers are steeped in hot water for several minutes before being strained and consumed. Tinctures are prepared by steeping the herb in alcohol or vinegar to extract its active compounds.

Dosage: The appropriate dosage of agrimony can vary depending on factors such as age, health status, and the specific preparation being used. It's important to follow the recommended dosage on the product label or consult with a qualified herbalist or healthcare professional for personalized guidance.

How to Use: Agrimony tea, tincture, or poultice is typically taken orally or applied topically. It's often consumed to soothe gastrointestinal issues, such as indigestion and diarrhea, or used externally to treat skin conditions.

Side Effects: Agrimony is generally considered safe for most people when used in moderate amounts. However, some individuals may experience allergic reactions or gastrointestinal upset. It may also interact with certain medications or have adverse effects in individuals with certain health conditions. It's important to use agrimony under the guidance of a healthcare professional and to discontinue use if any adverse effects occur.

Alfalfa:

Definition: Alfalfa, scientifically known as Medicago sativa, is a flowering plant in the pea family native to Asia but cultivated worldwide. It's primarily grown as fodder for livestock, but it has also been used in traditional medicine for its potential health benefits.

Ingredients: Alfalfa contains various bioactive compounds, including vitamins (such as vitamin A, vitamin C, and vitamin K), minerals (including calcium, magnesium, and potassium), amino acids, and phytoestrogens. These compounds are believed to contribute to the herb's medicinal properties, including its potential as a nutritive tonic, diuretic, and hormone balancer.

How to Prepare: Alfalfa is typically consumed as sprouts, herbal tea, or in supplement form (such as capsules or tablets). To make tea, dried alfalfa leaves are steeped in hot water for several minutes before being strained and consumed.

Dosage: The appropriate dosage of alfalfa can vary depending on factors such as age, health status, and the specific preparation being used. It's important to follow the recommended dosage on the product label or consult with a qualified herbalist or healthcare professional for personalized guidance.

How to Use: Alfalfa sprouts, tea, or supplements are typically taken orally. It's often consumed as a dietary supplement to support overall health and well-being, as well as to promote kidney health and hormone balance.

Side Effects: Alfalfa is generally considered safe for most people when consumed in moderate amounts. However, some individuals may experience allergic reactions or digestive upset. It may also interact with certain medications or have adverse effects in individuals with certain health conditions, such as autoimmune diseases or hormone-sensitive conditions. Pregnant or breastfeeding individuals should consult with a healthcare professional before using alfalfa supplements. It's important to use alfalfa under the guidance of a healthcare professional and to discontinue use if any adverse effects occur.

Ashwagandha:

Definition: Ashwagandha, scientifically known as Withaniasomnifera, is a small shrub native to India, the Middle East, and parts of Africa. It has a long history of use in Ayurvedic medicine for its potential health benefits, particularly for its adaptogenic properties.

Ingredients: Ashwagandha root contains various bioactive compounds, including alkaloids (such as withanolides), steroidal lactones, and flavonoids. These compounds are believed to contribute to the herb's medicinal properties, including its potential as an adaptogen, anti-inflammatory, and immune-modulating agent.

How to Prepare: Ashwagandha is typically consumed as a powdered root, herbal tea, tincture, or in supplement form (such as capsules or tablets). To make tea, dried ashwagandha root is steeped in hot water for several minutes before being strained and consumed.

Dosage: The appropriate dosage of ashwagandha can vary depending on factors such as age, health status, and the specific preparation being used. It's important to follow the recommended dosage on the product label or consult with a qualified herbalist or healthcare professional for personalized guidance.

How to Use: Ashwagandha powder, tea, tincture, or supplements are typically taken orally. It's often consumed to support stress management, promote relaxation, and boost overall vitality and well-being.

Side Effects: Ashwagandha is generally considered safe for most people when used in moderate amounts. However, some individuals may experience mild side effects such as gastrointestinal upset or drowsiness. It may also interact with certain medications or have adverse effects in individuals with certain health conditions, such as autoimmune diseases or thyroid disorders. Pregnant or breastfeeding individuals should consult with a healthcare professional before using ashwagandha supplements. It's important to use ashwagandha under the guidance of a healthcare professional and to discontinue use if any adverse effects occur.

Astragalus:

Definition: Astragalus, scientifically known as Astragalus membranaceus, is a flowering plant native to China and Mongolia but also found in other parts of Asia. It has been used for centuries in traditional Chinese medicine for its potential health benefits, particularly for its immune-enhancing properties.

Ingredients: Astragalus root contains various bioactive compounds, including polysaccharides, saponins (such as astragalosides), flavonoids, and amino acids. These compounds are believed to contribute to the herb's medicinal properties, including its potential as an adaptogen, immunomodulator, and anti-inflammatory agent.

How to Prepare: Astragalus is typically consumed as a powdered root, herbal tea, tincture, or in supplement form (such as capsules or tablets). To make tea, dried astragalus root slices are simmered in water for several minutes before being strained and consumed.

Dosage: The appropriate dosage of astragalus can vary depending on factors such as age, health status, and the specific preparation being used. It's important to follow the recommended dosage on the product label or consult with a qualified herbalist or healthcare professional for personalized guidance.

How to Use: Astragalus powder, tea, tincture, or supplements are typically taken orally. It's often consumed to support immune function, promote vitality, and enhance overall well-being.

Side Effects: Astragalus is generally considered safe for most people when used in moderate amounts. However, some individuals may experience mild side effects such as gastrointestinal upset or allergic reactions. It may also interact with certain medications or have adverse effects in individuals with certain health conditions, such as autoimmune diseases or diabetes. Pregnant or breastfeeding individuals should consult with a healthcare professional before using astragalus supplements. It's important to use astragalus under the guidance of a healthcare professional and to discontinue use if any adverse effects occur.

Goldenseal:

Definition: Goldenseal, scientifically known as Hydrastis canadensis, is a perennial herb native to North America. It has a long history of use in traditional Native American medicine and later in folk medicine for its potential health benefits.

Ingredients: Goldenseal root contains various bioactive compounds, including alkaloids (such as berberine and hydrastine), flavonoids, and volatile oils. These compounds are believed to contribute to the herb's medicinal properties, including its potential as an antimicrobial, anti-inflammatory, and immune enhancer.

How to Prepare: Goldenseal is typically consumed as an herbal tea, tincture, or in supplement form (such as capsules or tablets).

To make tea, dried goldenseal root or leaves are steeped in hot water for several minutes before being strained and consumed.

Dosage: The appropriate dosage of goldenseal can vary depending on factors such as age, health status, and the specific preparation being used. It's important to follow the recommended dosage on the product label or consult with a qualified herbalist or healthcare professional for personalized guidance.

How to Use: Goldenseal tea, tincture, or supplements are typically taken orally. It's often used to support immune function, promote digestive health, and soothe inflammation.

Side Effects: Goldenseal is generally considered safe for most people when used in moderate amounts. However, some individuals may experience mild side effects such as gastrointestinal upset or allergic reactions. It may also interact with certain medications or have adverse effects in individuals with certain health conditions, such as high blood pressure or pregnancy. It's important to use goldenseal under the guidance of a healthcare professional and to discontinue use if any adverse effects occur.

Hops:

Definition: Hops, scientifically known as Humulus lupulus, is a perennial climbing vine native to Europe, Asia, and North

America. It is primarily known for its use in brewing beer but has also been used historically in traditional medicine for its potential health benefits.

Ingredients: Hops flowers contain various bioactive compounds, including bitter acids (such as humulone and lupulone), essential oils, flavonoids, and polyphenols. These compounds are believed to contribute to the herb's medicinal properties, including its potential as a sedative, relaxant, and digestive aid.

How to Prepare: Hops is typically consumed as an herbal tea, tincture, or in supplement form (such as capsules or tablets). To make tea, dried hops flowers are steeped in hot water for several minutes before being strained and consumed.

Dosage: The appropriate dosage of hops can vary depending on factors such as age, health status, and the specific preparation being used. It's important to follow the recommended dosage on the product label or consult with a qualified herbalist or healthcare professional for personalized guidance.

How to Use: Hops tea, tincture, or supplements are typically taken orally. It's often used to promote relaxation, relieve anxiety, and support sleep.

Side Effects: Hops is generally considered safe for most people when used in moderate amounts. However, some individuals may experience mild side effects such as drowsiness, gastrointestinal upset, or allergic reactions. It may also interact with certain medications or have adverse effects in individuals with certain health conditions, such as depression or hormone-sensitive conditions. It's important to use hops under the guidance of a healthcare professional and to discontinue use if any adverse effects occur.

Kelp:

Definition: Kelp refers to several species of large brown algae belonging to the Laminariales order. It is commonly found in underwater forests along rocky coastlines around the world. Kelp has been used for centuries in various cultures, particularly in East Asia, for its nutritional and medicinal properties.

Ingredients: Kelp is rich in various nutrients, including iodine, vitamins (such as vitamin K, vitamin C, and B vitamins), minerals (including calcium, magnesium, and potassium), antioxidants, and fiber. These nutrients are believed to contribute to the seaweed's potential health benefits, including its role in thyroid function, bone health, and immune support.

How to Prepare: Kelp is typically consumed dried, powdered, or in supplement form (such as capsules or tablets). It can also be used in cooking, particularly in soups, salads, and stir-fries. Kelp supplements are available in various forms, including powdered extracts, tablets, and liquid extracts.

Dosage: The appropriate dosage of kelp can vary depending on factors such as age, health status, and the specific preparation being used. It's important to follow the recommended dosage on the product label or consult with a qualified healthcare professional for personalized guidance.

How to Use: Kelp supplements are typically taken orally with water. They can be consumed as part of a daily nutritional regimen to support overall health and well-being. Kelp can also be incorporated into recipes as a flavorful and nutritious ingredient.

Side Effects: While kelp is generally considered safe for most people when consumed in moderate amounts, excessive intake of iodine-rich foods or supplements, including kelp, can lead to thyroid dysfunction or iodine toxicity. Some individuals may also be allergic to seaweed and experience allergic reactions. Pregnant or breastfeeding individuals should consult with a healthcare professional before using kelp supplements. It's important to use kelp under the guidance of a healthcare professional and to discontinue use if any adverse effects occur.

Cat's Claw:

Definition: Cat's claw, scientifically known as Uncaria tomentosa, is a woody vine native to the Amazon rainforest and other parts of Central and South America. It has been used for centuries in traditional medicine by indigenous peoples for its potential health benefits.

Ingredients: Cat's claw contains various bioactive compounds, including alkaloids (such as oxindole alkaloids and quinovic acid glycosides), polyphenols, and other phytochemicals. These compounds are believed to contribute to the herb's medicinal properties, including its potential as an immune enhancer, anti-inflammatory, and antioxidant.

How to Prepare: Cat's claw is typically consumed as an herbal tea, tincture, or in supplement form (such as capsules or tablets). To make tea, dried cat's claw bark or leaves are steeped in hot water for several minutes before being strained and consumed.

Dosage: The appropriate dosage of cat's claw can vary depending on factors such as age, health status, and the specific preparation being used. It's important to follow the recommended dosage on the product label or consult with a qualified herbalist or healthcare professional for personalized guidance.

How to Use: Cat's claw tea, tincture, or supplements are typically taken orally. It's often used to support immune function, reduce inflammation, and promote overall well-being.

Side Effects: Cat's claw is generally considered safe for most people when used in moderate amounts. However, some individuals may experience mild side effects such as gastrointestinal upset or allergic reactions. It may also interact with certain medications or have adverse effects in individuals with certain health conditions, such as autoimmune diseases or bleeding disorders. Pregnant or breastfeeding individuals should consult with a healthcare professional before using cat's claw supplements. It's important to use cat's claw under the guidance of a healthcare professional and to discontinue use if any adverse effects occur.

Feverfew:

Definition: Feverfew, scientifically known as Tanacetum parthenium, is a perennial herb native to Europe but also found in other parts of the world. It has a long history of use in traditional medicine, particularly in European folk medicine, for its potential health benefits.

Ingredients: Feverfew contains various bioactive compounds, including sesquiterpene lactones (such as parthenolide), flavonoids, and volatile oils. These compounds are believed to contribute to the herb's medicinal properties, including its potential as an anti-inflammatory, analgesic, and migraine prophylactic.

How to Prepare: Feverfew is typically consumed as an herbal tea, tincture, or in supplement form (such as capsules or tablets). To make tea, dried feverfew leaves and flowers are steeped in hot water for several minutes before being strained and consumed.

Dosage: The appropriate dosage of feverfew can vary depending on factors such as age, health status, and the specific preparation being used. It's important to follow the recommended dosage on the product label or consult with a qualified herbalist or healthcare professional for personalized guidance.

How to Use: Feverfew tea, tincture, or supplements are typically taken orally. It's often used to alleviate headaches, including migraines, and to support overall well-being.

Side Effects: Feverfew is generally considered safe for most people when used in moderate amounts. However, some individuals may experience mild side effects such as gastrointestinal upset or allergic reactions. It may also interact with certain medications or have adverse effects in individuals with certain health conditions, such as bleeding disorders or pregnancy. It's important to use feverfew under the guidance of a healthcare professional and to discontinue use if any adverse effects occur.

Ginseng:

Definition: Ginseng refers to several species of perennial plants belonging to the Panax genus, including Panax ginseng (Asian ginseng) and Panax quinquefolius (American ginseng). Ginseng has been used for centuries in traditional medicine, particularly in East Asia, for its potential health benefits.

Ingredients: Ginseng root contains various bioactive compounds, including ginsenosides, polysaccharides, and peptides. These compounds are believed to contribute to the herb's medicinal properties, including its potential as an adaptogen, immune enhancer, and cognitive booster.

How to Prepare: Ginseng is typically consumed as a powdered root, herbal tea, tincture, or in supplement form (such as capsules or tablets). To make tea, dried ginseng root slices are simmered in water for several minutes before being strained and consumed.

Dosage: The appropriate dosage of ginseng can vary depending on factors such as age, health status, and the specific preparation being used. It's important to follow the recommended dosage on the product label or consult with a qualified herbalist or healthcare professional for personalized guidance.

How to Use: Ginseng powder, tea, tincture, or supplements are typically taken orally. It's often used to support energy levels, enhance cognitive function, and promote overall well-being.

Side Effects: Ginseng is generally considered safe for most people when used in moderate amounts. However, some individuals may experience mild side effects such as insomnia, gastrointestinal upset, or headaches. It may also interact with certain medications or have adverse effects in individuals with certain health conditions, such as high blood pressure or diabetes. Pregnant or breastfeeding individuals should consult with a healthcare professional before using ginseng supplements. It's important to use ginseng under the guidance of a healthcare professional and to discontinue use if any adverse effects occur.

Chickweed:

Definition: Chickweed, scientifically known as Stellaria media, is an annual herbaceous plant native to Europe but naturalized in many other parts of the world. It's often considered a common weed but has been used historically in traditional medicine for its potential health benefits.

Ingredients: Chickweed contains various bioactive compounds, including flavonoids, saponins, mucilage, and vitamins (such as vitamin C). These compounds are believed to contribute to the herb's medicinal properties, including its potential as a demulcent, anti-inflammatory, and mild diuretic.

How to Prepare: Chickweed is typically consumed as an herbal tea, infusion, or in fresh salads. To make tea, dried chickweed leaves and flowers are steeped in hot water for several minutes before being strained and consumed. It can also be used topically as a poultice or infused oil for skin conditions.

Dosage: The appropriate dosage of chickweed can vary depending on factors such as age, health status, and the specific preparation being used. It's important to follow the recommended dosage on the product label or consult with a qualified herbalist or healthcare professional for personalized guidance.

How to Use: Chickweed tea, infusion, or fresh leaves are typically taken orally. It's often used to soothe inflammation, support digestion, and promote overall well-being. Topically, chickweed can be applied to the skin to alleviate itching, irritation, or minor wounds.

Side Effects: Chickweed is generally considered safe for most people when consumed in moderate amounts. However, some individuals may experience allergic reactions or gastrointestinal upset. It may also interact with certain medications or have adverse effects in individuals with certain health conditions. Pregnant or breastfeeding individuals should consult with a healthcare professional before using chickweed supplements. It's important to use chickweed under the guidance of a healthcare professional and to discontinue use if any adverse effects occur.

Cleavers:

Definition: Cleavers, scientifically known as Galium aparine, is a herbaceous annual plant native to Europe, North America, Asia, and Australia. It has a long history of use in traditional medicine for its potential health benefits.

Ingredients: Cleavers contains various bioactive compounds, including iridoid glycosides, flavonoids, tannins, and mucilage.

These compounds are believed to contribute to the herb's medicinal properties, including its potential as a diuretic, lymphatic tonic, and mild astringent.

How to Prepare: Cleavers is typically consumed as an herbal tea, infusion, or in fresh salads. To make tea, dried cleavers leaves and stems are steeped in hot water for several minutes before being strained and consumed. It can also be used topically as a poultice or infused oil for skin conditions.

Dosage: The appropriate dosage of cleavers can vary depending on factors such as age, health status, and the specific preparation being used. It's important to follow the recommended dosage on the product label or consult with a qualified herbalist or healthcare professional for personalized guidance.

How to Use: Cleavers tea, infusion, or fresh leaves are typically taken orally. It's often used to support lymphatic drainage, promote urinary tract health, and soothe inflammation. Topically, cleavers can be applied to the skin to alleviate itching, irritation, or minor wounds.

Side Effects: Cleavers Is generally considered safe for most people when consumed in moderate amounts. However, some individuals may experience allergic reactions or gastrointestinal upset. It may also interact with certain medications or have adverse effects in individuals with certain health conditions. Pregnant or breastfeeding individuals should consult with a healthcare professional before using cleavers supplements. It's important to use cleavers under the guidance of a healthcare professional and to discontinue use if any adverse effects occur.

Eucalyptus:

Definition: Eucalyptus refers to a genus of flowering trees and shrubs, primarily native to Australia but also found in other parts of the world. Eucalyptus essential oil, extracted from the leaves of certain species, has a long history of use in traditional medicine for its potential health benefits.

Ingredients: Eucalyptus essential oil contains various bioactive compounds, including eucalyptol (cineole), terpenes, and flavonoids. These compounds are believed to contribute to the oil's medicinal properties, including its potential as an expectorant, decongestant, antiseptic, and anti-inflammatory.

How to Prepare: Eucalyptus essential oil can be used in aromatherapy, diffused in the air, or diluted and applied topically to the skin. It can also be added to steam inhalations or chest rubs to help relieve respiratory symptoms.

Dosage: The appropriate dosage of eucalyptus essential oil can vary depending on factors such as age, health status, and the specific application being used. It's important to follow the recommended dosage on the product label or consult with a qualified aromatherapist or healthcare professional for personalized guidance.

How to Use: Eucalyptus essential oil can be used aromatically, topically, or internally, depending on the intended application. It's often used to alleviate respiratory congestion, soothe sore muscles, promote relaxation, and support overall well-being.

Side Effects: Eucalyptus essential oil is generally considered safe for most people when used appropriately. However, it can be toxic if ingested in large amounts and should not be applied directly to the skin without proper dilution. Some individuals may experience allergic reactions or respiratory irritation when exposed to eucalyptus oil. It's important to use eucalyptus oil with caution, especially around children and pets. Pregnant or breastfeeding individuals should consult with a healthcare professional before using eucalyptus oil. If any adverse effects occur, discontinue use and seek medical attention.

Black Cohosh:

Definition: Black cohosh, scientifically known as Actaea racemosa (formerly Cimicifuga racemosa), is a perennial herb native to North America. It has a long history of use in traditional Native American medicine and later in folk medicine for its potential health benefits, particularly for women's health.

Ingredients: Black cohosh root contains various bioactive compounds, including triterpene glycosides (such as actein and cimicifugoside), phenolic acids, and flavonoids. These compounds are believed to contribute to the herb's medicinal properties, including its potential as a hormone-balancing agent and its ability to relieve menopausal symptoms.

How to Prepare: Black cohosh is typically consumed as a powdered root, herbal tea, tincture, or in supplement form (such as capsules or tablets). To make tea, dried black cohosh root is steeped in hot water for several minutes before being strained and consumed.

Dosage: The appropriate dosage of black cohosh can vary depending on factors such as age, health status, and the specific preparation being used. It's important to follow the recommended dosage on the product label or consult with a qualified herbalist or healthcare professional for personalized guidance.

How to Use: Black cohosh powder, tea, tincture, or supplements are typically taken orally. It's often used by women to support hormonal balance, relieve menopausal symptoms such as hot flashes and night sweats, and promote overall well-being.

Side Effects: Black cohosh is generally considered safe for most people when used in moderate amounts. However, some individuals may experience mild side effects such as gastrointestinal upset or allergic reactions. It may also interact with certain medications or have adverse effects in individuals with certain health conditions, such as liver disease or hormone-sensitive conditions. Pregnant or breastfeeding individuals should consult with a healthcare professional before using black cohosh supplements. It's important to use black cohosh under the guidance of a healthcare professional and to discontinue use if any adverse effects occur.

Blessed Thistle:

Definition: Blessed thistle, scientifically known as Cnicusbenedictus, is an annual or biennial herb native to the Mediterranean region but also found in other parts of Europe, Asia, and North Africa. It has been used historically in traditional medicine for its potential health benefits, particularly for digestive and liver health.

Ingredients: Blessed thistle contains various bioactive compounds, including sesquiterpene lactones (such as cnicin), flavonoids, tannins, and essential oils. These compounds are believed to contribute to the herb's medicinal properties, including its potential as a digestive tonic, appetite stimulant, and liver tonic.

How to Prepare: Blessed thistle is typically consumed as an herbal tea, tincture, or in supplement form (such as capsules or tablets). To make tea, dried blessed thistle leaves and flowers are steeped in hot water for several minutes before being strained and consumed.

Dosage: The appropriate dosage of blessed thistle can vary depending on factors such as age, health status, and the specific preparation being used. It's important to follow the recommended dosage on the product label or consult with a qualified herbalist or healthcare professional for personalized guidance.

How to Use: Blessed thistle tea, tincture, or supplements are typically taken orally. It's often used to support digestion, stimulate appetite, and promote liver health.

Side Effects: Blessed thistle is generally considered safe for most people when used in moderate amounts. However, some individuals may experience mild side effects such as gastrointestinal upset or allergic reactions. It may also interact with certain medications or have adverse effects in individuals with certain health conditions, such as hormone-sensitive conditions or bleeding disorders. Pregnant or breastfeeding individuals should consult with a healthcare professional before using blessed thistle supplements. It's important to use blessed thistle under the guidance of a healthcare professional and to discontinue use if any adverse effects occur.

THE END

www.ingramcontent.com/pod-product-compliance
Lightning Source LLC
Chambersburg PA
CBHW081843250726
48659CB00008B/2594